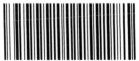
NAVIGATING
NURSING

NAVIGATING NURSING

A PRACTICAL GUIDE FOR THE
NOVICE NURSE FROM A TO Z

YASHAMIKA SHORT, MSN, RN-BC

NAVIGATING NURSING
Published by Purposely Created Publishing Group™
Copyright © 2020 Yashamika Short

Printed in the United States of America

ISBN: 978-1-64484-134-1

Special discounts are available on bulk quantity purchases by book clubs, associations and special interest groups. For details email: sales@publishyourgift.com or call (888) 949-6228. *For information log on to:* www.PublishYourGift.com

*To new graduate nurses
wanting to know what's next.*

TABLE OF CONTENTS

INTRODUCTION

As a nurse with 19 years of experience, I still remember my first job and first year working as a nurse. That experience has never left me. I had two of the best preceptors. My first nursing job was at a Level 1 Trauma Center in a Surgical Trauma Intensive Care Unit (ICU). I don't remember being scared of the environment because I worked as a certified nursing assistant (CNA) while in nursing school. However, I was not accustomed to the complexity of the patients, communicating with physicians, operation of the equipment, and being 100 percent accountable for the patient's care. I remember assessing my patient and looking over at my preceptor who had this look of "what are you doing and why are you doing it in that order?" I worked with nurses who wanted me to succeed and probably a few who didn't, but my goal was to learn and give the best care possible to my patients.

My journey in nursing has taken me on a lot of different paths, but my current path has been one of the most fulfilling. In the last ten years, I've worked with new graduate nurses who are eager about nursing and excited to care for patients, which is refreshing, but they truly have no idea what lies ahead of them just like I didn't. Coordinating a nursing residency program has allowed me to learn, share, and guide the transition from nursing student to graduate nurse to novice nurse. They've laughed, cried, felt doubtful, stressed, questioned their profession and themselves, but through it all, they conquered their fears, overcame obstacles, and succeeded. My hope is that this book gives you REAL and PRACTICAL insight into what to expect when you enter the nursing profession and lets you know that what you are feeling and thinking is not abnormal. Those thoughts and feelings are there to give you something to anticipate, prepare for, and conquer. Having a clearer vision of what lies ahead allows you to have tools in your toolbox when complex situations arise. When you are aware, you face your challenges with a greater sense of confidence. After all, your first year sets the tone for what comes next whether good, bad, or indifferent.

A

ASSESSMENT

Assessment is what the nurse bases his or her nursing care and interventions on. It determines the need to notify the physician or anyone on the interdisciplinary team. This is a skill you should be extremely efficient in. An assessment should be done at the beginning of every shift, with any change in your patient's condition, and when your patient leaves and returns from a procedure. To do an assessment, a nurse should always have a stethoscope, unless you have superpowers that allow you to hear heart, lung, and bowel sounds from afar.

An assessment sets the baseline of your day. It identifies what's going on with the patient and gives you the ability to recognize a change and identify trends. It's the catalyst to the care you provide the patient. Don't ever get too busy that you omit this step. It seems like Nursing 101; however, there are many nurses who fail to complete this task. Can't believe it, right?

"My patient's condition can deteriorate at the drop of a hat, and I've learned to be diligent with assessment, assessment, assessment."

—New Graduate Nurse

ACCOUNTABILITY

You are the gatekeeper of the patient. Everyone else on the interdisciplinary team comes and goes throughout the day, but you are the constant for your shift (8 hours, 12 hours, etc.). Because you are the most consistent aspect of the care your patient receives, I find that nurses often get the brunt of the mistreatment and distrust from the patients or family. My belief is that they feel you are the one thing that they can possibly control. I don't think nursing school gives you a clear depiction of this.

As the nurse, most questions are funneled through you. There have been many times I've encouraged patients or families to ask the doctor questions when they round or visit, but on most interactions, the patient or family will not ask the doctor questions but, as soon as the doctor leaves, will turn to the nurse and ask questions. Go figure! The nurse should be held responsible for the nursing care provided or lack thereof.

ADVOCATE

Because you are the gatekeeper, you must fight for what's best for your patients. Sometimes that means stepping outside of your comfort zone to do so. If you can't advocate for yourself, how can you advocate for the patient? It's a big responsibility, but the world expects it. Nursing is considered one of the most trusted professions.

As reported by the American Organization of Nurse Executives (AONE), nurses were ranked as the most trusted profession in 2017, according to the annual Gallup poll on honesty and ethical standards. Nurses have topped the list of 22 professions for the past 16 years.[1]

"Patient advocacy is such a huge part of patient care in my unit, and it's very important to me."

—New Graduate Nurse

REFLECTIONS

REFLECTIONS

_____

_____

_____

_____

_____

_____

_____

_____

_____

_____

_____

_____

_____

_____

_____

REFLECTIONS

B

BOARD OF NURSING (BON)

Know what is expected of you from your state's BON. Know your Nurse Practice Act. Know the American Nurse Association Code of Ethics.

Each state's expectations and rules are different, so know what standards you are being held to. Know how and when to renew your license based on where you live. You should also know what education requirements are expected in order to maintain a license in "good standing" and how many continuing education (CE) hours are needed. Keep a folder of your continuing education certificates in the event you are audited by your state's BON. Having your certificates is also helpful as proof of professional development during your performance evaluation. The BON determines whether or not you keep or lose your license. Having an understanding of your hospital and state's Peer Review and Safe Harbor process (if applicable to your state) is important as well.

REFLECTIONS

REFLECTIONS

REFLECTIONS

REFLECTIONS

_____

_____

_____

_____

_____

_____

_____

_____

_____

_____

_____

_____

_____

_____

_____

C

COMMUNICATION

Communication is the cornerstone of our profession. You are always communicating with someone about something. Whether it's the patient, the family, the doctor, or the interdisciplinary team, you are required to communicate with others. You must be able to articulate your thoughts. Sit down and analyze your strengths and weaknesses and practice your delivery. Think about it and provide your answers in the table: What would you consider your communication style and why? Identify a situation where communicating became difficult and how you responded. Practice using Situation, Background, Assessment, Recommendation (SBAR) or Team Strategies and Tools to Enhance Performance and Patient Safety (TeamSTEPPS) if your organization uses that process. The Agency for Healthcare Research and Quality (AHRQ) has an abundance of resources for TeamSTEPPS.[2]

"Proper communication can literally save lives."

—New Graduate Nurse

"It's never safe to assume. Communication and being thorough is most important for the patient's safety."

—New Graduate Nurse

How would you identify your communication style?

_____

_____

_____

_____

My communication:

STRENGTHS	CHALLENGES

Describe a difficult conversation and how you responded:

_____

_____

_____

_____

_____

_____

_____

_____

_____

_____

_____

_____

_____

_____

_____

CONFLICT

Conflict is a natural process. Analyze how you currently deal with conflict. Are you the person who deals with the issue or who avoids the issue? How do you feel when you deal with conflict versus not dealing with conflict? What tools do you think you will need to have difficult conversations with doctors, patients, and families?

Running away from conflict can cause your patients harm. You may be thinking she wants me to argue with everyone and be confrontational. No, not at all. I want you to pick your battles, but when it comes to patient safety, you must confront the situation to keep your patients safe.

You may encounter situations involving patient assignments, inappropriate medication dosages, or patient status changes. Always use terms that people hear and respond to. Don't just state your feelings. Unfortunately, most people really don't care how you feel. Using words like overwhelmed and tired don't hold much weight because the person you are talking to probably feels the same way, so they are thinking "join the club." Using the acronym CUS (Concerned, Uncomfortable, and Safety) works great in situations where you are trying to convey the severity of the situation. For example, I'm concerned that the patient's blood pressure is 80/50, and it makes me uncomfortable to care for her on this unit. For the safety of the patient, she needs to transfer to a higher level of care.[3]

A family member tells you they don't want you to be the nurse who is assigned to his or her relative. How would you respond?

The patient flirts with you and asks you about your personal life? How do you respond?

Those are examples of situations you may experience, so you should have some planned responses in your toolbox to use when these situations arise. If you stay ready, you never have to get ready!

How do you deal with conflict?

_____

_____

_____

_____

What tools do you think you will need to prevent being afraid of having difficult conversations?

_____

_____

_____

_____

Come up with your own CUS statements:

_____

_____

_____

_____

CONFIDENCE

Confidence develops over time, but don't worry—it will come. Be confident in who you are because you are a NURSE. You passed the NCLEX. Show people how to treat you. Don't think that because you are the "low man or woman" on the totem pole you don't deserve respect. You can disagree with a person and still be treated with respect. You know more than you give yourself credit for.

When processing events, situations, or interventions; map out what you know before you approach your preceptor. If you still have questions or are unsure, approach your resource letting him or her know that you know step one, step two, and maybe step four but get confused on step three. By identifying what you know, you build your confidence, and your preceptor will likely acknowledge that and assist you in thinking through the missing process. Remember going to your preceptor or resource without any real information, processing, or insight will not help build your confidence or critical thinking skills.

When you exude confidence or assurance, it puts the patient and family at ease. Asking questions doesn't take away from your confidence; in fact, it displays your humility and lets others know you want the best for them.

Confidence also sets the tone for who is facilitating the care. Knowing the top five to ten diagnoses and medications that are common to your area will make you feel more confident about the care you provide as well. It will take at least a year before you begin to feel "completely confident" in your nursing skill and judgment.

"I have to work on my confidence! I know the information and have the skills, so I have to start trusting myself and my instincts."

—New Graduate Nurse

REFLECTIONS

_____

_____

_____

_____

_____

_____

_____

_____

_____

_____

_____

_____

_____

_____

_____

_____

REFLECTIONS

REFLECTIONS

D

DOCUMENTATION

Documentation is an important part of your job and role. Documentation helps doctors determine the care the patient needs. Documentation determines reimbursement for the doctor and hospital. Documentation paints the picture of the patient's care. Anyone reviewing your charts should be able to visualize what you did for that patient during your shift. Ask your preceptor or create your own documentation checklist that identifies what and where items need to be documented. Your documentation should be clear and concise. Know what is expected of you in your department and legally.

As the saying goes, "If you didn't document it, it wasn't done." By visiting the remediation section of your BON website, you will find reasons why detailed documentation is important. There are plenty of examples of how the lack of documentation negatively impacted the care of the patient.

DOCTORS

Let's just start off by saying that doctors are human, and they put their pants on one leg at a time like everyone else. Don't give them more power than they deserve. They should be viewed as your biggest ally and collaborator. After all, you both need each other to provide great care to the patient. The nurse-doctor relationship is like an arranged marriage. You don't meet or talk to each other until you work together at the bedside, which is *too late*. The late interaction makes for a rocky start to the relationship. The relationship should be initiated while both are in their respective school training. This could help remove the stigma and fear. To help chip away at that fear, think about and ask yourself what's the worst that could happen if I call or if I don't call the doctor for assistance? There are only a few options if you call: they may hang up in your face, ignore the call, scream, answer the call and be very pleasant, etc. But remember all those things mentioned are things you've endured before whether from your guardian, spouse, partner, or friend. Guess what? You survived, so you will survive this encounter and the others that will follow. So don't let fear keep you from doing the right thing. Identify and write down what would keep you from calling (perceived versus realistic) and escalating the patient's care to the doctor. Then identify what's the worst that could happen if you don't call and escalate. Then weigh the consequences on both sides to see which has a heavier outcome.

Remember why you became a nurse. Most often that reason is to care for others. When you don't make the call, you have become selfish and no longer are thinking about the patient but about *yourself* and what's going to happen or how they will respond to you if you call. It's not about you; it's about the patient.

"I feel communication is very important on my unit. The more interaction I get with the physician, the more comfortable I get."

—New Graduate Nurse

What will/could keep me from calling the doctor?

_____

_____

_____

_____

What are my fears?

_____

_____

_____

_____

Analyze your fears, perceived versus realistic.

PERCEIVED	REALISTIC

What solutions are available to address my fears?

_____

_____

_____

_____

DEATH

Death happens more times than not depending on your unit or area of specialty. Be aware of how you feel as well as how the family feels. Don't say you understand because even if you have had a family member or friend die, what you felt may not be what that family is feeling. Don't let silence during this time make you uncomfortable. In fact, appreciate it. Most times, silence is the best thing, and your presence with the family is the icing on the cake. Take time to process what happens after the death and your shift. It's okay to cry. After all, you are human too.

After your patient's transition, be sure to acknowledge your thoughts and feelings. It's okay to ask for a few minutes to examine what happened. It's also okay to think about it after leaving work. After all, you are human.

Death is something everyone is going to face, but the most important aspect is the support we provide our patients and families and then the support we receive as nurses. Become familiar with your chaplains. They can provide significant support even if the patient does not follow a particular religion or spirituality. Chaplains can also be of service to you.

"A memorable experience is a patient's family member saying 'thank you' and giving hugs after their loved one passed."

—New Graduate Nurse

DELEGATION

Know what your BON says about delegation and your role as the nurse. Know what you can and cannot delegate and to whom you can delegate tasks. If you are working on a unit that employs Licensed Vocational Nurses (LVN), be familiar with their scope of practice. As a new nurse, you will attempt to do everything yourself because that reassures you that it's done, but you have to work smarter and not harder. You must use your resources to make a better work environment and to decrease burnout. Trying to do everything yourself will lead to resentment. Remember nursing is a 24-hour job. You don't have to get it all done in one shift, but don't make a habit of leaving work for your peers either. Don't be the nurse that, regardless of your patient assignment or acuity of your patients, leaves work for the next shift because you were so "busy." Always having an excuse about why you didn't call the doctor, draw the labs, take the patient to MRI, or perform other tasks is not acceptable.

Always have three things you can delegate if someone asks if you need help. Don't let your mind convince you that those who offered help don't have time to help because they have their own patients. You're projecting your feelings on those individuals. If they asked you how they can help, then they are extending themselves for your benefit, so give them something to do.

"It's usually hard for me to delegate because I feel responsible for my workload, and I feel like I need to be able to handle things on my own."

—New Graduate Nurse

"I have difficulty delegating when I think I can do it."

—New Graduate Nurse

REFLECTIONS

REFLECTIONS

REFLECTIONS

E

EXPECTATIONS

What are your expectations from your preceptor, peers, leadership, or organization? If your preceptor has not given you expectations, you need to ask. You also need to be clear what you want from them and your leaders. Ask your leader what's their leadership style. You can't meet a goal if you don't know what you are reaching for or being measured against. You should never leave a meeting during orientation with your educator, preceptor, or manager without goals, challenges to improve, or identification of your strengths.

What are your expectations?

_____

_____

_____

_____

What do you expect from your peers?

_____

_____

_____

_____

What do you expect from your preceptor?

_____

_____

_____

_____

What do you expect from your organization?

_____

_____

_____

_____

ERRORS

You may make mistakes; some may be small and others may be significant, but the key is to recognize and admit to making them and learn from them. Don't cover them up and act like they didn't happen. Being open and transparent about your imperfections yields understanding and empathy. Own up to it. If you ever happen to make an error, you will likely not make that same error again. It creates a learning opportunity and is a humbling experience for you. The key to preventing errors is following ALL the steps in ALL sequences ALL the time. Don't let others (doctors, nurses, patients, families, or peers) rush you into doing something you don't feel comfortable doing.

ESCALATION

Escalation is defined as "to involve someone more important or higher in rank in a situation or problem."[4]

Asking or requesting something when you feel like you didn't get a solution whether it's a return phone call, an inappropriate order, or an inappropriate assignment may be the first level of escalation. Remember that you have not fully escalated up the chain of command until you have a resolution or solution to your questions or concerns. If you are escalating up the chain of command on the physician side, you should simultaneously escalate up the chain of command on the nursing side.

Food for thought: You call the doctor regarding the patient's blood pressure (BP). The doctor doesn't call you back. You don't sit on it and wait until they round, but you call again. You have to identify when or how long to wait before you make the next call. An Attending Physician (head MD) once said if it's an emergency, give the doctor five minutes max. And if it's important, give the doctor 15 to 30 minutes before you phone again or escalate up the chain of command. Remember don't waste your time calling the same person for a solution if he or she is not willing to give you one. Work smart not hard! You should not call any provider more than two times if you are not getting a response. After the second call and no response, you should move to the next person in charge. Continuing to call the same person is a waste of your time and delays care for the patient.

REFLECTIONS

REFLECTIONS

REFLECTIONS

_____

_____

_____

_____

_____

_____

_____

_____

_____

_____

_____

_____

_____

_____

_____

_____

REFLECTIONS

F

FRIENDS

As they say, you spend most of your time at work, and as a nurse, that's typically 12 hours a day. Your friendships will change. Most of your friends work traditional hours and days while you work 12 hours, holidays, and possibly every other weekend. Most of your time off will come while they are at work, which will change your friendship dynamics. By no means am I saying you will no longer have friends, but your relationships will look different. Most will feel like, "You only work three days a week, so why are you tired?" They may not realize you are mentally and physically drained from dealing with people and their families who are experiencing a significant situation in their lives. So it's best to have a friend at work or at least in healthcare who will understand what and how you feel when you vent or complain about your day without making you feel like a bad person because you didn't have a great experience with your patient or their family that day.

"I would change that I have to work so many weekends."

—New Graduate Nurse

FAMILY

You will now become the "go-to person" for answers to all the ailments in your family. Time with them will change as well. You will have to plan or think of alternative days to celebrate for holiday time because you may be at work.

One of my graduate nurses said, "Mother's Day has always been a special time with my mom, and I've never had to think about whether I was going to spend it with her until I started working as a nurse." So know there will be some compromises when it comes to the time you get to spend with family and friends.

When will you celebrate Thanksgiving, Christmas, New Year's Eve, or your special holidays if you are working?

What are some options for celebrating the holidays?

_____

_____

_____

_____

FEEDBACK

Feedback is pivotal in your growth and development, but you must be able to receive it. Talk with your preceptor or educator about how you would like to receive feedback whether good or bad. Do you like to hear the good first, and then the bad or challenges? Do you prefer the sandwich effect: good, challenges, good? Have that conversation because it's important that you are able to hear it and grow. This should be established on day one of meeting your preceptor. Also, ask your preceptor how they would like to receive feedback about their performance from your standpoint. Remember this is a relationship, and both sides have to establish likes and dislikes.

How do you like to receive feedback?

_____

_____

_____

_____

FLOATING

Floating is the "F" word in nursing. It's when a nurse has to leave his or her home unit to work in another unit. When nurses find out that they have to float to another unit, you often see the not so pleasant side of that person. Going to another unit is all in one's perspective. One thing for sure, nursing care doesn't change. Regardless of what unit or floor you are working, you will call or intervene about the concerns: change in blood pressure or heart rate, decrease in urine output, change in level of consciousness, or change in lab values. What does change is who you are notifying, so try to approach floating as a day that your scenery will be different, but the care expectations are the same. Also, don't show up to a unit saying what you don't know or can't do but instead advertise your strengths utilizing the statements below.

This is the skill set that I have . . .

_____

_____

_____

_____

This is what I'm validated or competent to do . . .

_____

_____

_____

_____

Perspective makes your day easier.

_____

_____

_____

_____

REFLECTIONS

REFLECTIONS

REFLECTIONS

_____

_____

_____

_____

_____

_____

_____

_____

_____

_____

_____

_____

_____

_____

_____

G

GRACE

Give yourself space to be imperfect. This is not a career where you will come in knowing it all at once. Don't be so hard on yourself. If you were a 4.0 student, don't expect to be a 4.0 nurse, at least not within the first year. There is a HUGE learning curve with this profession. Regardless of how much you know from the books, you have to be able to apply it, which comes with time and experience.

As the quote says, "Every expert was a beginner." Enjoy the ride.

*"Biggest challenge has been everything.
I feel like I don't know anything, and I feel overwhelmed constantly. I don't love it. I have anxiety every day before I have to go back for another shift."*

—New Graduate Nurse

GRAY

If you think in black and white, there will be some challenges within your transition. Nursing has a lot of gray areas. If you bring experience from a previous career like accounting or engineering where x=x all the time, there will be some challenges in changing your thought process to be open, flexible, and fluid. Be open to what's between x because in healthcare there is usually something there but not as apparent. No two patients with the same diagnosis will present the same, have the same medications, and do what the textbook describes. However, the beauty of the gray gives you the opportunity to act as the sleuth and solve the mystery. The fun part.

"The patients give me great memories, but that feeling of knowing how to care for them and what to do for them at every turn gives me the greatest sense of accomplishment."

— **New Graduate Nurse**

"One thing I definitely learned was that nursing is unpredictable."

—**New Graduate Nurse**

REFLECTIONS

_____

_____

_____

_____

_____

_____

_____

_____

_____

_____

_____

_____

_____

_____

_____

_____

_____

REFLECTIONS

REFLECTIONS

REFLECTIONS

H

HONEYMOON

This is when you feel like all in the world is great. You've graduated nursing school, passed NCLEX, and now have a job. Well, that feeling changes, and your emotions will be up and down as you transition through your first year as well as throughout your nursing career. In fact, there will be times when you question why you chose this profession. This is probably a question you will ask yourself frequently throughout your career, not just the first year. Always refer back to why you became a nurse. It's a hard profession, but it's worth it.

"I feel so motivated. I'm motivated to spark change and make a difference in healthcare."

—New Graduate Nurse

"The hardest part of nursing to adjust to was that every patient doesn't want to be helped."

—New Graduate Nurse

What is your nursing WHY?

_____

_____

_____

_____

_____

_____

_____

_____

_____

_____

_____

_____

_____

_____

_____

_____

REFLECTIONS

REFLECTIONS

_____

_____

_____

_____

_____

_____

_____

_____

_____

_____

_____

_____

_____

_____

_____

_____

_____

REFLECTIONS

REFLECTIONS

I

INTUITION

According to the Merriam Webster online dictionary, intuition is "a natural ability or power that makes it possible to know something without any proof or evidence." If you've heard of mother's intuition meaning that a mother knows when something is going on with her child even though the child has not mentioned anything or she has not actively seen something, then you will understand how intuition works. Well, nurses have that too. It's a feeling that you get based on what you see or hear in regard to your patient. Sometimes you can't put the "what" into words, but it's there. That feeling will never lead you wrong. In fact, *tap into it*. That feeling will grow as your career and experience grows, giving you words and actions to articulate to physicians, patients, and families.

True story: A nurse had a patient who was nonverbal. While reviewing the patient's labs, the nurse recognizes that the patient's hemoglobin/hematocrit (H&H) decreased, but the patient presented with no signs and symptoms of concern. The nurse felt the patient just didn't look right. The nurse called the physician and articulated her concerns. The physician authorized the nurse to draw labs and transfer the patient to a higher level of care. Once the patient arrived at the Intermediate Unit, the lab results were back. The patient's H&H had decreased significantly, accompanied with blood in their stool. The patient was transferred to the ICU for a gastrointestinal bleed.

Trust your intuition!

INTERDISCIPLINARY

The interdisciplinary team consists of doctors, respiratory therapists, social workers, case managers, clinical managers, physical therapists, speech therapists, and occupational therapists, etc. All of these professionals play a key part in the care of the patient. Get to know them by name, their role, and their impact. Establishing those relationships makes taking care of the patient easier.

"Ensuring patients with emotional needs get with social work, patient with pain management get evaluated by doctors, and patients with financial concerns get help from case managers is important. I spend a lot of time using my communication or interpersonal skills to get needed interprofessional team members around my patients to ensure quality patient care."

—New Graduate Nurse

Identify who is on the interdisciplinary team. What is their actual role? I included a few members below. Who else can you think of?

Interdisciplinary team:

Case manager role/responsibilities:

_____

_____

Social worker role/responsibilities:

_____

_____

Risk manager role/responsibilities:

_____

_____

_____ role/responsibilities:

_____

_____

_____ role/responsibilities:

_____

_____

REFLECTIONS

REFLECTIONS

REFLECTIONS

_____

_____

_____

_____

_____

_____

_____

_____

_____

_____

_____

_____

_____

_____

_____

_____

REFLECTIONS

_____

_____

_____

_____

_____

_____

_____

_____

_____

_____

_____

_____

_____

_____

_____

_____

J

JOURNEY

Run your race. Your transition will not be like your peers' or friends'. Even if your orientation is shorter or longer than your peer's, it does not guarantee that either of you will be a better nurse than the other. Also, know when to throw the towel in. If you find yourself in an area or unit that is weighing on you emotionally and physically outside of the "normal" feeling of inadequacies that come with being a new nurse, then it's time to re-evaluate that area or unit. How do you differentiate the "normal" versus "abnormal?" Well, the abnormal is when you can't leave the work at work. When work plays on your psyche. All nurses wonder after their shift if they did this or that, but when you are not able to shut that voice off, then it could potentially be a problem. One way to leave work at work is to establish a landmark or place where you will stop thinking about work. For example, you can say once I park my car in the garage at home, I will no longer think about what I did and did not do at work. That establishes boundaries and clear thoughts. Your place can be anywhere or anytime but just establish one. Identify and write down two places or times that you can identify as your stopping point for leaving work at work.

> *"One of the biggest challenges is the fear that*
> *I am forgetting something important,*
> *that I haven't been taught yet."*

—New Graduate Nurse

My landmark to no longer think about work is:

1. _____   2. _____

JOB FIT

A lot of new nurses long to work in the Intensive Care Unit (ICU), but it's not for everyone. No, I'm not saying, like others, that you need to work on a medical/surgical unit to get your skills before you become an ICU nurse. I worked in an ICU right out of nursing school. I think the ability to work in the ICU is an individualized decision based on the person. When looking for your first job, consider what area or body system in nursing school (during clinical) you enjoyed the most. Regardless of what happened, how they treated you, what the patient said or did to you, what area were you still excited to go back to the next morning? That's likely where you should work.

I've noticed new nurses focus on which hospital they want to work at but not the unit. The unit is where your time is spent. That first year is precious and long, so being in the area of choice makes a HUGE difference. Don't let others, including your professors, convince you that you can work anywhere for a year. You can, but believe me, it's not easy or fun. I've seen quite a few new nurses leave their first job within six months of starting because it's not where their heart or interest is. Don't be bamboozled or swayed. *Get hired for the unit and not the hospital.* If you don't get the unit at the hospital you desire, it's okay to go where your desired unit is. Once you've acquired the experience of working in that unit, come back to the hospital you originally desired.

True story: A nursing student came to our Nurse Residency Program Open House event and was very excited about working in the operating room (OR). She was so excited that even as a nursing student, she attended the local OR nursing organization meetings. To my surprise, she accepted a position at our hospital in a different area than the OR. Guest what? After 8 months, she resigned from our facility and went to another hospital to work in the OR. To this day, I tease her about her choice, and she reminds me that I told her so and that she should have listened.

Write a list of the areas you are interested in and make a list of the pros and cons. Write what role the nurse plays in patient care in that area. What are the pros and cons of the patient population? How long is the commute time?

Organization I'm considering:

_____

Commute? If so, how long?

_____

Specialty:

_____

PROS	CONS

Nurse's role/responsibilities:

_____

Shift: day or night? How will working this shift impact my social/family life? How will I adjust to the change?

_____

_____

_____

_____

Organization I'm considering:

_____

Commute? If so, how long?

_____

Specialty:

_____

PROS	CONS

Nurse's role/responsibilities:

_____

_____

_____

_____

Shift: day or night? How will working this shift impact my social/family life? How will I adjust to the change?

_____

_____

_____

_____

Organization I'm considering:

_____

Commute? If so, how long?

_____

Specialty:

_____

PROS	CONS

Nurse's role/responsibilities:

_____

_____

_____

_____

Shift: day or night? How will working this shift impact my social/family life? How will I adjust to the change?

_____

_____

_____

_____

REFLECTIONS

_____

_____

_____

_____

_____

_____

_____

_____

_____

_____

_____

_____

_____

_____

REFLECTIONS

REFLECTIONS

K

KINDNESS

Treat people as you want to be treated. This principle is so simplistic and basic but not often followed. At times, we don't treat our work family, our patients, or our patient's family kind. If everyone kept the patient at the center, it would decrease some of the personal things that are brought into play. The example that comes to mind is the nurse–patient care assistant (PCA) relationship. If you ask the PCA to help the patient get dressed and the PCA gives you attitude or the PCA asks the nurse to help bathe the patient and she or he gives attitude, kindness is not being displayed. The question is why the attitude. People need to look at it as you're not helping me, but you're helping the patient. I dressed myself this morning and was able to bathe myself, so this is not a personal request but a request for the patient. Think about some things you think might get in the way of you being kind. Now that you've thought of those things, what are some ways to change that thought to make it more about the patient?

> *"Work feels like an attachment of home.*
> *I feel welcomed and invited."*

—New Graduate Nurse

What might get in the way of me being kind?

_____

_____

_____

_____

What can I do to redirect those feelings or attitudes?

_____

_____

_____

_____

REFLECTIONS

REFLECTIONS

_____

_____

_____

_____

_____

_____

_____

_____

_____

_____

_____

_____

_____

_____

_____

_____

_____

REFLECTIONS

REFLECTIONS

L

LATERAL VIOLENCE

Lateral violence is often classified as bullying, incivility, and aggression. According to the American Nurse Association (ANA), bullying is defined as "repeated, unwanted, harmful actions intended to humiliate, offend, and cause distress in the recipient."[5]

For as long as I can remember there has always been this saying: "Nurses eat their young." I could never understand why. You are there to help make the shift go easier, allow for staff to enjoy vacations, and decrease the calls asking nurses to come in to work on their days off. Oftentimes, new nurses are treated as outsiders by experienced nurses who become territorial like they have something to prove. It's like we want new nurses to prove themselves. For what? It doesn't always lead to a more productive or more efficient nurse.

Lateral violence can be as simple as someone rolling their eyes while you are talking to them, purposely ignoring you doing handoff report, not intentionally helping when you ask for assistance, gossiping about you to your peers, and withholding information.

I feel like lateral violence starts in nursing school with the student-professor relationship. A lot of instructors make it their mission to give you a hard time when they should be providing an encouraging learning environment. Every nurse had or knows someone who had a nursing instructor treat them and likely a few others like they had a point to prove. The profession is hard enough when dealing with people who are experiencing a significant life-changing event, and adding difficult coworkers to the mix can sometimes be unbearable for a new nurse.

As with any bully, you should address the behavior of the aggressor and set boundaries and expectations. Pick the appropriate time to discuss the situation. If you don't feel comfortable talking with that person alone, then ask for a mediator (manager, educator, or fellow peer) to be present. Never accept bad treatment because once you do, it can become your new normal. That causes people to feel resentful, hate the profession, and leave nursing.

Check out the article *Teaching Cognitive Rehearsal as a Shield for Lateral Violence: An Intervention for Newly Licensed Nurses* by Martha Griffin. This article provided some practical solutions when dealing with lateral violence.[6]

REFLECTIONS

REFLECTIONS

REFLECTIONS

M

MINDFULNESS

Be in the moment, which is easier to say and harder to do in the clinical environment. Nurses are good, but at times, we let our abilities block our rationale. Let's paint the picture. Often, call lights are on, patient monitors are beeping, phone calls from families, patients, and doctors are coming during handoff report, and peers are conversing about non-nursing situations. Nurses are at the medication station having side conversations. We, unfortunately, accept this as the norm. There must be time set aside to be in the moment with minimal distractions. Mindfulness is especially critical during medication administration, procedures, receiving orders, and other tasks. During medication administration, one way to decrease conversation with family or patients is to set the boundaries prior to administration. Maybe you can say, "At this time, I would like to talk only about your medications. After I've given you your medication, I will answer and discuss any other concerns you may have." You could use that statement for different things besides medication administration and add other statements that fit the moment.

Write:

What other times during your shift should be sacred?

_____

_____

_____

_____

What are some things you could do to be mindful during critical times?

_____

_____

_____

_____

MEDICATIONS

You should know the top five to ten medications that are given in your area or unit. Knowing that information gives you confidence, keeps you safe, and makes you more efficient.

Having this information makes you a resource for the patients, families, and physicians. Follow whatever your hospital policy says about medication administration. Don't cut corners. Trust the process with your high-risk medication two-person identifiers. Don't get complacent and do walk by checks. Walk by is when the nurse walks by and quickly looks at the medication, doesn't check the order, doesn't look to see if the medication was given to the right person, or other important factors. Be the nurse that follows all the checks and balances.

REFLECTIONS

_____

_____

_____

_____

_____

_____

_____

_____

_____

_____

_____

_____

_____

_____

_____

REFLECTIONS

REFLECTIONS

N

NURSE

You have chosen the best profession in the whole world. I'm a little biased, however, what other career do you know of where you can do so many things? Teachers are the only profession that probably comes close to the options nurses have and the number of nursing specialties available. The sky is the limit. (See the list below for some examples.) So don't become a grouchy nurse because you have options!

▶ Legal interest: Legal Nurse Consultant

▶ Advanced Mid-level Provider: Acute Care Nurse Practitioner

▶ Primary Care Provider: Adult, Geriatric, Psychiatric, and/or Family Nurse Practitioner

▶ Forensics: SANE Nurse (Sexual Assault Nurse Examiners)

▶ Education: Nurse Educator/College Faculty

▶ Computers: Nurse Informatics

▶ Anesthesia: CRNA (Certified Registered Nurse Anesthetists)

▶ Community Assistance: Public Health/ Occupational Health

▶ Family and Resource Engagement: Case Manager

▶ Administration: Clinical Manager, Director, Chief Nursing Officer (CNO), Chief of Operations (COO), Chief Executive Officer (CEO)

▶ Sales: Pharmaceutical Representative

▶ Check out American Nurse Credentialing Center (ANCC), where you can find certification information for a variety of nursing specialties, including the specialists listed above (www. nursingworld.org).

▶ Also look into your specialty organizations like the Medical-Surgical Nursing Certification Board or the Board of Certification for Emergency Nursing, just to name a few (www.nursingcenter. com).

NIGHT SHIFT

Traditionally, new nurses work the night shift. It's not for everyone. Night shift has its pros and cons. Most times, it's approximately $10,000 more a year. Don't let others convince you that night shift is easier because it's not. Sometimes your sickest patients are admitted during this time. Think about how people's behavior become riskier as the sun sets. Outside of that, you have to be diligent with your health and well-being working nights. Try black out curtains to sleep and make sure you have a decent meal at night because most times the cafeteria at your hospital will not have the healthiest options available. A lot of people rely on coffee and energy drinks to get through. There's no judgment from me, but think of how you will maintain. Typically it will take you two days to recover when you are off. So take all those things into consideration if you are on a unit or at a hospital that lets you self-schedule your workdays.

Write:

How will you maintain? (What will your meal consist of? When will you eat? When will you sleep? What about your social life?) Bring protein snacks, eat less carbs, and bring lunch.

_____

_____

_____

What's your game plan for getting food during your shift?

_____

_____

_____

_____

What is the game plan for sleeping?

_____

_____

_____

_____

REFLECTIONS

REFLECTIONS

REFLECTIONS

REFLECTIONS

_____

_____

_____

_____

_____

_____

_____

_____

_____

_____

_____

_____

_____

_____

0

ORIENTATION

This is probably one of the most important things about your transition. This will guide how you practice and assimilate into your area or unit. You, along with your preceptor, must be on the same page and have an open relationship. You must be able to communicate what you need and expect from your preceptor. Never leave a meeting or discussion with your preceptor, manager, or educator with unspecific feedback even if they say you are doing great. That type of feedback is very generic with no substance. Always ask for specifics and goals for the next encounter. See how important feedback is? It's so important I had to mention it again.

Nurses are creatures of muscle memory. We do so many things simultaneously that it's hard to identify one thing we do and tell someone about it. If you don't believe me, think about this. This can apply to nursing students or new nurses. If I asked you what you do all day or what your day consists of, can you tell me? Think about it for a few minutes. I know the answer is no. We can't articulate our day, but we can identify what is missing because we are typically trying to find the missing piece to the picture of what's going on with our patients. Because of this inability to articulate what's missing, nurses have a hard time giving feedback on performance. So, as the orientee, you must know your expectations and goals. I often ask the preceptor or clinical coaches how I can grade or assess an orientee's skill or clinical application if I don't know what I am looking for or measuring them against.

> *"My preceptor can be condescending."*
>
> **—New Graduate Nurse**

> *"If I could change something, it would be more time with my preceptors to go over my performance, how I am doing, and what is expected of me."*
>
> **—New Graduate Nurse**

OVERCOMPLAIN

Nurses overcomplain and under report. Nurses tend to tell each other their gripes and issues but don't voice those issues to the person who can fix the issue or provide a solution. Nurses get in the mode of "I'm not going to say anything because nothing is going to change." That mentality leads to increased stress, burnout, and dissatisfaction. To combat those things, nurses should use the power that they have. That power may look different in different organizations, but nurses must use it. Nurses are typically the biggest workforce in the hospital setting but sometimes have the smallest voices. That power involves completing surveys about their work environment, reporting systems, or processes to identify unacceptable behavior from doctors, peers, or other healthcare providers. Letting others know what you expect is what changes the culture or environment, not silence and complacency. There is power in numbers. You may silence one, but you can't silence and ignore 1,000.

REFLECTIONS

REFLECTIONS

REFLECTIONS

_____

_____

_____

_____

_____

_____

_____

_____

_____

_____

_____

_____

_____

_____

_____

P

PATIENT CARE ASSISTANTS (PCA)

PCAs are individuals who are there to assist the nurse and help care for the patient. For a long time, there has been a power struggle between the nurse and the PCA. The PCA thinks the nurse is not doing anything but giving meds, and the nurse may feel the PCA should do all the "hard" work like turning the patients, giving baths, providing toileting assistance, and checking vital signs. There should be collaboration between the two roles with the patient being the center focus. I feel people lose sight of that. I think nurses, especially new nurses, miss the opportunity to forge the relationship based on assumptions of their role. Some new nurses think they don't have to do certain things like cleaning up poop or changing sheets because they're the nurse. Sorry, but that's not true. Those things are a part of your job, and you should be doing them too. You have the license; therefore, the patient is your responsibility. The key to this dynamic is communication and inclusion. If you give your PCA report on the patients that you share and discuss the plan of care for the day, that will take you a long way. They will feel like they are a part of the team and not just your assistant.

Food for thought: Regardless of the size or makeup of the unit, patient care assistants always have more patients than the nurse.

"I have difficulty delegating to PCAs."

—New Graduate Nurse

"I learned to delegate to PCAs. They are great assets!"

—New Graduate Nurse

POLICIES AND PROCEDURES

Be familiar with your organization's policies and guidelines. Know your hospital's and unit's standards of care. Most nurses practice based on what they were taught rather than what's expected. Verify that what your preceptor is teaching you is what's expected. It's not okay for you to say you didn't know the policy.

PRIORITIZING

Make sure you create dialogue around this pivotal component of your orientation. Prioritizing and time management will be one of your biggest challenges in developing your nursing practice. In my opinion, what makes this difficult is that most preceptors don't teach this skill but rather "teach" by demonstration. They don't walk and talk you through how they determine what patient to see first or show you how to cluster your care, so that you are utilizing your time efficiently. Also, if your preceptor gets called away, you should be going with them. They should not be leaving you to finish the task while they go handle another situation. Splitting the care in that manner does not show you how to readjust when your care gets interrupted.

Food for thought: You and the preceptor receive a report together. After report, the preceptor explains which patient you will see first, second, etc., and why. As time goes on in your orientation, the pendulum shifts. After report, your preceptor will ask you to prioritize which patient you will see first and why. When that shift happens, it is based on what you and your preceptor decide. Teaching in that manner allows your preceptor to model and teach the behavior, then give you the opportunity to apply it.

"My biggest challenge has been establishing a routine for my day. It seems there is always something new that kicks me out of sync."

—New Graduate Nurse

PERFORMANCE EVALUATION

Performance evaluations typically happen annually in most organizations. If this is your first career or job, then there will be a learning curve. Typically, during this timeframe, your organization will likely have you identify your strengths, weaknesses, goals (short and long-term), and accomplishments from the year. This is your time to shine and highlight all you've done or been recognized for. Comment cards from peers, leadership, families, and patients are great to have for this evaluation. The proof is in the pudding. Keeping records of your continuing education certificates shows continued development and learning. Precepting nursing students or other new graduate nurses, participating in hospital or unit committees, and acting as the charge nurse are leadership skills that should be highlighted. This evaluation typically comes with a merit (monetary) increase, so you want to convince your leaders of your worth. Having documentation of your development is how you identify your value and worth.

REFLECTIONS

REFLECTIONS

REFLECTIONS

REFLECTIONS

Q

QUESTIONS

Continue to ask questions. A nurse who doesn't ask questions is a nurse who shouldn't be practicing. No one always has the answers. Don't let others make you feel less than for asking questions because they will try to make you feel less qualified. Questions help with critical thinking and application.

Questions keep you safe!

REFLECTIONS

REFLECTIONS

REFLECTIONS

_____

_____

_____

_____

_____

_____

_____

_____

_____

_____

_____

_____

_____

_____

_____

_____

R

RESILIENCE

According to the Merriam Webster Dictionary, resilience means "an ability to recover from or adjust easily to misfortune or change."[7] Resilience is being heavily researched and written about in the nursing community. According to the Nurse Executive Center Advisory Board, in order for leaders to build a more resilient nursing workforce, they must address violence and point-of-care safety threats in the healthcare setting. Nurses feel they have to compromise care delivery. Staff bounces from traumatic experiences to other care activities with no time to recover, and new technology, responsibilities, and care protocols cause nurses to feel "isolated in a crowd."[8] As a nurse, once you walk in the hospital, you are on stage. I always joke with my peers and new graduate nurses that nurses should have an Academy Award. Once you walk into the hospital and onto your unit, what you felt or what was going on personally no longer matters. You have to step out of your world. Your beliefs and biases can no longer exist. Your day consists of dealing with ethical challenges that you may not agree with. As a nurse, you are constantly giving and rarely being deposited into, sometimes feeling like an ATM. When you have moments of "thank you" or "you did a great job" or "you took such great care of me," you need to treasure those times because they don't happen often enough. In order to keep coming back, you must find ways to decompress.[9]

"I've learned that I need to get enough sleep and food to effectively provide the best care for my patients."

—New Graduate Nurse

"Memorable moments so far have been when patients and family members tell me how great I was in taking care of them. It's happened quite a few times, and it really makes me see why I chose this as my career."

—New Graduate Nurse

REFLECTIONS

REFLECTIONS

REFLECTIONS

REFLECTIONS

S

STRESS

It's part of the journey. The key is identifying when you are stressed, what causes you stress, and tools to work through the stress. You will feel overwhelmed but know you are not the first nurse to feel that way nor will you be the last. Find ways to let go whether that's through exercise, reading, running, or other hobbies or activities that help you redirect your mind from work. What typically happens is that new nurses are extremely stressed since they are learning a new profession and the complexity of healthcare. However, once new nurses complete orientation, they tend to work overtime for whatever reason, which adds additional stress. My suggestion is to not do overtime (OT) during the first three to six months after completing orientation; just get used to being a nurse, establishing a routine, and perfecting your craft. Nurses tend to pick up extra shifts for financial reasons whether it's paying for a wedding, a new house, new car, or vacation. We look at getting those items by completing additional shifts. In no way am I counting your coins or passing judgment because I've done it myself. But those extra shifts come with consequences especially if you are already burned out or overworked. So before working OT, do a self-assessment of where you are on the "burnedometer."

If you acquire paid time off (PTO) or vacation days, use them whether it's a staycation or an elaborate getaway. You owe it to yourself, your patients, and your family. Don't be that nurse who says I haven't taken a vacation in five years. That's not healthy. Everyone needs a reprieve.

"I'm learning to cope with the stress of the job and slow process of becoming proficient."

—New Graduate Nurse

"I'm working to decrease stress and decompress after work in following days off."

—New Graduate Nurse

How does your mind and body respond to feeling overwhelmed?

_____

_____

_____

_____

How do you work through those feelings?

_____

_____

_____

_____

What activities help relieve your stress?

_____

_____

_____

_____

Find out what resources your organization offers (i.e., gym memberships, licensed counselors, etc.)

_____

_____

_____

_____

REFLECTIONS

REFLECTIONS

_____

_____

_____

_____

_____

_____

_____

_____

_____

_____

_____

_____

_____

_____

_____

_____

REFLECTIONS

REFLECTIONS

T

TIME

Time is the nurse's kryptonite. Whenever a nurse says, "I can't do something," a majority of the time, it's driven by "I don't have time" or the perception of "I don't have time." More times than not, the time is there, but your ability to recognize that is based on the many tasks you foresee completing. When "I don't have time" creeps into your day, ask yourself is it an emergency or is it something I have to do now? Based on your answer to those questions, determine the next question. Is it my perception, or have I realistically allotted myself time to complete the task? What and who are my resources to create that time? Your answers will guide your movement and actions. Going through that process will help chip away at that kryptonite.

"I'm not used to constantly completing task after task after task without stopping."

—New Graduate Nurse

REFLECTIONS

REFLECTIONS

REFLECTIONS

U

UNDERSTANDING

Put yourself in your patient's family's shoes. Don't get caught up in the "drama" or non-essential information given to you in report or discussed on the unit about the patients or your peers. Whether you believe it or not, hearing the non-essential changes the lens from which you view your patients and peers. Sometimes the background is much deeper than the revealed. Develop your own understanding. A good video to watch that brings this home is *Empathy: The Human Connection to Patient Care* created and produced by the Cleveland Clinic. This video is available on YouTube.

"It's difficult at times to refrain from judgment. I've realized that I don't really know these people's stories, and I have no right to pass judgment. I need to maintain the same respect for all patients no matter the situation."

—New Graduate Nurse

REFLECTIONS

REFLECTIONS

REFLECTIONS

V

VIOLENCE

Unfortunately, violence has become more common in the workplace of healthcare providers. The National Crime Victimization Survey showed healthcare workers have a 20 percent higher chance of being the victim of workplace violence than other workers (Joint Commission, 2018). With fewer and fewer mental health facilities available and more patients presenting to the hospital with a medical diagnosis along with a mental health diagnosis, the perfect storm is created. Active shooters are another component that healthcare workers must take into account. There have been instances where an active shooter entered the hospital and caused harm. For that reason, anytime you enter on a unit, you should always survey the environment for potential hiding places and possible exits. Many organizations provide training on how to de-escalate situations. There are states that consider violence to a healthcare worker a criminal offense. So please check with your state to see what laws they have in place.[10]

Write:

What are my state, city, and or county laws for assaulting a healthcare worker?

_____

_____

_____

_____

REFLECTIONS

REFLECTIONS

REFLECTIONS

_____

_____

_____

_____

_____

_____

_____

_____

_____

_____

_____

_____

_____

_____

_____

_____

REFLECTIONS

W

WHY

You will be a two-year-old all over again. If you have a kid or have been around toddlers, they tend to ask "why" quite frequently as they figure out the world around them. That will be you. Wanting to know the why is what makes great nurses. There will be times your preceptor or peer will ask you to do something, and you have no idea why or how, but you don't ask follow-up questions prior to performing the task. Once the task is performed and it's done incorrectly, there is a problem. So always ask for clarification when you are unsure. Not doing so, as I mentioned earlier, is being selfish and thinking about you and how you will feel if your peer or preceptor feels the question is not warranted. Remember, it's not about you, but it's about the patient. The WHY makes us call the family, the doctor, talk with the patient, and lean on our peers. The WHY will never go away. Don't let it go away and don't let someone take it away.

WINS

Celebrate the small wins. There's so much to grasp and learn in your first year you will feel like I'm not doing this right, or I'm never going to get it at times. But during every shift you should aim to do tasks better than you did the shift before, the hour before, or the minute before. So write those small wins down regardless of how simple they may seem. Doing so boosts your confidence and gives you a better picture of how you've grown from day one.

Examples of small wins:

▶ I charted before lunch time.

▶ I gave recommendations to the doctor.

▶ I clocked out on time.

▶ I got the IV on the first stick.

REFLECTIONS

REFLECTIONS

REFLECTIONS

REFLECTIONS

X

EXCITEMENT

This time in your life will come with many moments of excitement. Graduation from nursing school, passing NCLEX, searching for and securing a job, meeting new friends, and transitioning into a new profession with new responsibilities are all exciting. Take in every moment, the highs and the lows, because all those moments make you who you are.

> *"The thing I've liked most is seeing the positive results of my daily care."*
>
> **—New Graduate Nurse**

> *"I love getting to know my patients and being able to make a difference."*
>
> **—New Graduate Nurse**

REFLECTIONS

REFLECTIONS

REFLECTIONS

_____

_____

_____

_____

_____

_____

_____

_____

_____

_____

_____

_____

_____

_____

_____

_____

Y

YEAR

You will make it through the first year and the many years that follow. You may find yourself in another unit or specialty, but you will survive like others before you. Every nurse remembers their first year no matter how many they have under their belt. Remembering that first year makes all the years to follow that much sweeter. There's nothing like recognizing your growth. In fact, I challenge you to write yourself a letter at the beginning of your first year. The letter can be about what you think you will be doing in the years to follow, how you are feeling as a new graduate nurse, or what you would like to tell yourself in a year. After writing the letter, seal the envelope and place it somewhere you can retrieve it. Put a reminder on the calendar in your phone to open the letter a year from now. You will be amazed at what you thought and how your perspective has changed.

REFLECTIONS

REFLECTIONS

REFLECTIONS

Z

ZERO TOLERANCE

Have zero tolerance for accepting anything less than what's best for you and your career. Expect a great preceptor, a great orientation, a healthy work environment, feedback whether good or bad, accountability, to give great patient care, and a leader who develops you. Hold yourself accountable to get what is best for you and to provide those same expectations to your peers, patients, and future nurses that you will one day precept.

REFLECTIONS

REFLECTIONS

_____

_____

_____

_____

_____

_____

_____

_____

_____

_____

_____

_____

_____

_____

_____

_____

_____

REFLECTIONS

CLOSING

One of my favorite moments of working with new graduate nurses is witnessing the "light bulb moment" where it all comes together. I hope your light bulb came on quite a few times in your reading. Nursing is not easy, but I can't say it enough that it's worth it especially when you find your home or happy place in whatever your specialty may be.

Be great and welcome to the BEST profession in the world!

NOTES

1. American Hospital Association, January 10, 2018: https://www.aha.org/news/insights-and-analysis/2018-01-10-nurse-watch-nurses-again-top-gallup-poll-trusted-professions.

2. TeamSTEPPS® is an evidence-based teamwork system aimed at optimizing patient care by improving communication and teamwork skills among healthcare professionals, including frontline staff: https://www.ahrq.gov/teamstepps/index.html.

3. CUS Reference: Team Strategies and Tools to Enhance Performance and Patient Safety: www.ahrq.gov/teamstepps/instrutctor/essentials/pocketguide.html.

4. *Cambridge Dictionary*, *s.v.* "escalate," dictionary.cambridge.org/us/dictionary/English/escalate.

5. American Nurse Association: Violence, Incivility, and Bullying: https://www.nursingworld.org/practice-policy/work-environment/violence-incivility-bullying/.

6. Griffin, M. (2004). "Teaching Cognitive Rehearsal as a Shield for Lateral Violence: An Intervention for Newly Licensed Nurses." *The Journal of Continuing Education in Nursing* (35) 6,257–263.

7. *Merriam-Webster Dictionary,* s.v., "resilience," https://www.merriam-webster.com/dictionary/resilience.

8. Rebuild the Foundation for a Resilient Workforce: Best Practices to repair the cracks in the care environment. August 8, 2018, retrieved from https://www.advisory.com/research/nursing-executive-center/white-papers/2018/rebuild-the-foundation-for-a-resilient-workforce.

9. Check out "American Nurse Association: A Call to Action: Exploring Moral Resilience Toward a Culture of Ethical Practice" for information about moral resilience at https://www.nursingworld.org/~4907b6/globalassets/docs/ana/ana-call-to-action--exploring-moral-resilience-final.pdf.

10. The Center for Disease Control (CDC) has an educational module on workplace violence prevention for nurses at https://www.cdc.gov/niosh/topics/violence/training_nurses.html.

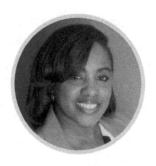

ABOUT THE AUTHOR

Yashamika Short, MSN, RN-BC, is a registered nurse certified in Nursing Professional Development with a clinical background in trauma and critical care. She holds a Master of Science in Nursing Education and has nineteen years of experience.

Yashamika currently works for a large hospital system as a Nurse Residency Coordinator. In 2016, she received the Good Samaritan Nurse Excellence Bronze Award and was nominated as employee of the year. She desires to leave a legacy in nursing and to encourage and enrich those coming after her.

While she enjoys teaching and mentoring nurses, in her spare time, she partakes in reading, traveling, and her newfound passion, gardening. She is also passionate about volunteering with organizations that give back to women and children such as I.C.O.N. Women's Organization and Keioko Davidson's Elementary Parent Teacher Association and living her life in full color.

Yashamika currently resides in Katy, Texas, with her husband and two children.

To connect, email her at yashamika.short@gmail.com or follow her on Instagram @yashamikashortRN

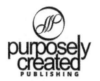

CREATING DISTINCTIVE BOOKS
WITH INTENTIONAL RESULTS

We're a collaborative group of creative masterminds
with a mission to produce high-quality books to position
you for monumental success in the marketplace.

Our professional team of writers, editors, designers,
and marketing strategists work closely together to ensure
that every detail of your book is a clear representation
of the message in your writing.

Want to know more?
Write to us at info@publishyourgift.com
or call (888) 949-6228

Discover great books, exclusive offers, and more at
www.PublishYourGift.com

Connect with us on social media

@publishyourgift